Liver Cleanse & Detox

14-Day Routine for Detoxing Your Body Using Foods
High in Nutrients and Herbal Remedies

Mitchell T. Theresa

Introducing the exclusive and captivating world of Mitchell T. Theresa. Immerse yourself in the timeless elegance and creativity that defines our brand. Experience the unparalleled craftsmanship and attention to detail that sets us apart. Discover the essence of sophistication and style with our exquisite collection.

Table of Contents

Preface

Greetings from a voyage of rejuvenation and self-discovery! Are you prepared to take the first steps toward your best possible health and wellbeing? Our bodies and minds frequently take the brunt of everyday stressors, pollution, and bad lifestyle choices in today's fast-paced environment. But have no fear—the transforming power of cleanse detox rests in the midst of the chaos, offering promise.

Imagine yourself as a more alive, vivacious version of yourself who exudes calmness within. This is something you can achieve, not some far-off dream. The cleansing detox movement is taking the health world by storm and providing a ray of hope for people looking to get well. People are becoming more aware of the significant advantages of cleaning their bodies and brains, whether they live in a busy city or a tranquil rural setting.

What precisely is cleanse detox, and why is it capturing so many people's interest? Fundamentally, cleansing detox is a holistic path to wellbeing rather than just getting rid of toxins from your body. You can access limitless energy and vitality by supporting mindfulness practices, feeding your body with nutrient-rich meals, and developing a closer relationship with your inner self.

Doubting the science of cleansing detox? Get ready to be in awe. Numerous advantages have been linked to detoxifying the body, according to research, including better digestion, better control over weight, and increased mood and mental clarity. You may activate your body's innate healing processes and restore your health by getting rid of dangerous pollutants and refuelling it with necessary nutrients.

Are you prepared to make the decision to start your liver cleanse and detox? Every stage of the process will be guided by our transformation roadmap. We've put together a thorough guide to help you reach your wellness objectives, from daily mindfulness exercises and self-care rituals to customized food plans and delectable recipes. Prepare to fuel your mind, body, and soul like never before.

Are you still unsure about starting a Liver cleanse & detox? Allow our inspirational testimonies to transform you. Hear from actual people who have personally benefited from cleansing detoxification. Their experiences, which range from successful weight loss to restored vitality and energy, are proof of the effectiveness of purification and rejuvenation.

Are you prepared to change the course of your life and live a vibrant, healthy existence? This is where your trip starts. You'll be equipped with all the knowledge and resources you need to start down the path to optimum health and wellbeing if you have our in-depth cleanse detox guide in hand. Bid farewell to exhaustion, tension, and stress — and welcome to a lively, invigorated version of yourself.

Remember this as you set out on your path to cleanse and detoxify: the options are virtually limitless. Liver cleanse & detox provides a route to change, whether your goal is to lose extra weight, increase your energy, or just get your life back. Accept the ride, have faith in the process, and get ready to reach your greatest potential.

Are you prepared to become the best version of yourself and join the Liver cleanse & detox movement? I cordially encourage you to start the change process right now. As your travel partner on this in-depth cleansing detox program, you'll experience self-realization, rejuvenation, and empowerment. Bid adieu to constraints and welcome to an endless life of energy and health.

To sum up, Liver cleanse & detox is a way of life, not just a fad. You can find the secrets to optimum health and vitality by supporting mindfulness practices, feeding your body with nutrient-rich meals, and developing a closer relationship with your inner self. Thus, why do you delay? Are you prepared to embark on this journey?

Introduction

In "Liver Cleanse & Detox," set off on a life-changing path to vibrant health and revitalized energy. Join acclaimed holistic wellness specialist Mitchell T. Theresa as she shares the keys to restoring your health and liver function.

Learn about the dramatic effects of a carefully designed liver cleanse program. This thorough guide gives you the tools to cleanse your body, rejuvenate your liver, and activate your body's natural healing capacity with step-by-step instructions and professional insights.

On a 14-day detoxification plan intended to eliminate toxins, promote liver regeneration, and boost energy levels, bid adieu to weariness, bloating, and sluggishness. This book provides you with all the tools you need to attain long-lasting wellness, from nourishing detox recipes to innovative lifestyle techniques.

Utilize nutrient-rich superfoods and evidence-based herbal treatments to optimize liver health and unleash the power of nature's remedies. "Liver Cleanse & Detox" provides a road map to restored energy and lifespan, regardless of the problems you're facing, such as persistent weight gain, abdominal problems, or chronic inflammation.

Take advantage of detoxification's life-changing effects as you set out to revitalize your body, mind, and soul. This book is the ideal guide to robust health, full of helpful hints, motivational success stories, and actionable guidance.

Thousands of people have already benefited from liver cleansing and detoxification; become one of them. With "Liver Cleanse & Detox," embrace wellness from the inside out and unleash your body's innate healing capacity. This is where your path to optimum health begins.

Chapter 1

Discover the Power of Liver Cleansing Foods and Natural Herbs for Optimal Health and Fitness

Chicory, scientifically known as Cichorium intybus

This plant known for its liver cleansing properties has brought vegetables like escarole or endive into the spotlight. The leaves serve dual purposes in the kitchen and for healing. Moreover, its dried root can be seen as a healthy alternative to coffee. Similar to a vegetable, preparing it is simple, and when combined with other ingredients that balance its bitterness, it can be used to make tasty and soothing salads with nutritional and healing benefits.

Exploring the Uses and Functions

Whether fresh or dried, it's best to use it before meals. The components in this product can boost appetite in both children and adults while also supporting digestive health. Thanks to its lactucopicrin, responsible for the bitter taste of chicory leaves, it also has a cholagogue effect, helping to empty the gall bladder and thus enhancing food digestion. It effectively purifies the liver and enhances its performance. Chicory is ideal for individuals dealing with gallbladder and liver issues as well as sluggish digestion.

With its gentle laxative effect, it helps with chronic constipation, while its mild diuretic effect can prevent fluid retention. Utilize dried chicory root as a coffee alternative, offering a caffeine-free digestive drink.

Effective ways to utilize Chicory

Utilize the freshly picked leaves in salads or to make fresh juice. The juice has a strong bitter taste but is very effective in boosting appetite. For preparing decoctions, use either fresh or dried root (2 teaspoons per glass). The primary can also be dried and ground for making a coffee alternative (dried, roasted, and raw). It can be used to maintain liquid form by taking 2 to 6 drops daily, divided into several doses.

Chicory Remedies

To make a digestive decoction, combine a cup of water with two teaspoons of chicory root and simmer for 5 minutes. Allow it to steep for ten minutes and then cool. Drinking 2 to 3 mugs of water every day before meals can help stimulate your appetite and improve digestion.

Recommendations for a Mindful Lifestyle

1.Starwest Wildcrafted Roasted Chicory Main Granules made from roasted chicory root

Starwest provides high-quality, wildcrafted chicory root granules that are roasted for easy preparation to create teas and decoctions for liver cleansing. Starwest is one of the top suppliers of organic and wildcrafted natural herbs in the galaxy. Preferences are fantastic and user-friendly.

Artichoke, scientifically known as Cynara scolymus

In the past, it was not highly valued as a therapeutic herb, but starting from the twentieth century, it has gained recognition as a remedy for liver cleansing and biliary disorders. Several of its compounds are found in pharmaceutical products that support liver health.

Exploring the Uses and Functions of Artichokes

Both the leaves and stem, whether fresh or dried, are effective in treating liver damage and biliary diseases, as well as protecting the liver from poisons. It truly enhances bile production and flow, supporting healthy digestion.

This treatment comes highly recommended for sluggish digestion and liver issues. Moreover, it acts as a diuretic, purifier, and aids in eliminating urea, making it beneficial for individuals with kidney issues. Artichoke is effective in reducing blood cholesterol levels.

Effective ways to utilize Artichokes

One common method to benefit from its medicinal properties involves consuming fresh artichoke heads. If you enjoy artichokes, you can also make fresh juice from the leaves. Remember to consume it right away as it's best within two hours. Infuse by adding 1 teaspoon of dried and chopped leaves per glass. Make the most of it by using tincture (1 teaspoon [6 milliliters] every 8 hours), ampoules (using the liquid extract), and pills (dried artichoke or powdered form).

Remedies for Artichokes

Alone

To ensure proper digestion of food, steep one teaspoon of leaves in a glass of boiling water. Let it steep for 10 minutes and then cool. Consume it approximately half an hour before your meals. Perhaps it's sweetened with sugar or honey.

Merged

Prepare a regulatory hepatic infusion by combining equal parts of liver-cleansing herbal ingredients boldo, artichoke, and thistle. Mix a teaspoon of the blend into each glass of boiling water and let it steep for 10 minutes. Enjoy it by drinking three mugs daily, approximately 30 minutes before meals.

Recommendations for a Mindful Lifestyle

Experience the benefits of wildcrafted artichoke capsules with Paradise Herbal's Artichoke Extract.

Paradise Herbs offers a premium full-spectrum artichoke leaf extract that is grown without the use of chemicals or pesticides. This unique low heat extraction method maintains all the fragile liver-cleansing therapeutic elements just as nature intended.

Boldo, scientifically known as Peumus boldus

The indigenous population of Chile, living in the Andes region, utilized boldo leaves to treat stomach and digestive issues. Today, it's a widely used remedy found in pharmacies and health food stores. This plant is highly regarded for its effectiveness in pharmaceuticals targeting gallbladder disorders.

Applications and Purpose.

This remedy is highly valued for its ability to protect the

liver and enhance bile production as well as promote gallbladder emptying. Boldo leaves are highly recommended for issues related to gallbladder function, like slow or challenging digestion, bloating, and bitter taste in the mouth, caused by gallbladder dysfunction. Moreover, it's a gentle yet powerful laxative that aids in combating chronic constipation.

Effective ways to utilize Boldo

Typically, dried and chopped boldo leaves are utilized to create infusions (one teaspoon per glass). However, it is often used in combination with other choleretic and cholagogue plants or laxatives. Moreover, it can be purchased in tablet form with recommended dosages provided by the manufacturer. Moreover, the components are derived from boldo bark and used in certain pharmaceuticals to treat liver and gallbladder conditions.

Boldo Treatments

Alone

For biliary dyspepsia infusion, steep a teaspoon of leaves

in a glass of boiling water. Let it steep for 10 minutes and then cool it down. Consume 3 mugs daily, approximately 30 minutes before eating.

Merged

Try this liver organ decongestant tea: mix together equal parts of boldo, fumitory, rosemary, dandelion, and anise for a cleansing herbal blend. Put two teaspoons of the mixture into a glass of boiling water. Let it steep for 10 minutes and then cool it down. For improved liver function, consume up to 3 cups before meals.

Recommendations for a Mindful Lifestyle.

Check out the Amazon Therapeutics Organic Boldo Tincture, made from wildcrafted boldo.

Experience the premium organic extract in a convenient tincture form for effortless consumption. Derived from the native vegetation of the Chilean and Peruvian mountains, Therapeutics Boldo tincture is a potent natural remedy for protecting and detoxifying the liver. Full-spectrum extracts are optimized for maximum effectiveness.

Milk thistle, scientifically known as Silybum marianum

Milk thistle is a liver-cleansing herb that is considered a wholesome food and natural herb. It grows wild throughout the USA and Europe.

Thistle thrives in Mediterranean temperate regions and has been utilized since ancient times. During the winter season, this vegetable is a common sight at Christmas gatherings in many places. The flavor is delicate, pleasant, and slightly bitter. While not particularly rich in nutrition, this ingredient contains other energetic components like silymarin and inulin, which contribute to its therapeutic properties.

Applications and Purpose

This remedy is highly effective for protecting and restoring the liver. It contains silymarin, which can regenerate damaged liver cells and reduce inflammation in liver tissue caused by toxins and bacteria. Milk Thistle is a great remedy for hepatitis and liver failure. It's also effective in addressing liver issues caused by insufficient bile secretion, like gallstones and biliary dyspepsia. These hepatoprotective leads can help ease symptoms associated with overeating, alcohol consumption, and drug abuse. On top of that, thistle boosts appetite, acts as a diuretic, has a mild laxative effect, and aids in lowering cholesterol levels due to its lipid-lowering properties. Moreover, it could be applied externally as an anti-inflammatory to help with sunburn and dermatitis.

Utilizing Milk Thistle to its full potential

Available in tinctures (1/4 to 1/2 teaspoon [1 to 2 milliliters] every 8 hours), water extracts (20 to 30 drops, two or three times a day), and dried and ground for making infusions. The capsules are finely ground and come with recommended dosages from the manufacturer. Furthermore, silymarin is derived from the fruits of milk thistle and is used in various liver medications.

Remedies with Milk Thistle

Standing alone

Brew a teaspoon to support a healthy liver. Add 5 thistle flowers to a glass of water and bring it to a boil for 2 minutes. Let it steep for five minutes and then cool it down. Consume two to three cups daily before meals to support optimal liver function.

Merged

Create a hepatoprotective tea by combining equal parts of liver-cleansing ingredients such as milk thistle, rosemary, and boldo. Use a teaspoon of the blend in a glass of boiling water, and let it steep for 10 minutes. Enjoy it as a pre-meal drink. This tea is great for soothing the liver after indulging in too much food.

Recommendations for a Mindful Lifestyle.

Discover the power of Omnibiotics Organic Milk Thistle Extract capsules.

Experience the power of Omnibiotics with its potent 4:1 milk thistle extract in a vegetarian capsule, free from synthetic ingredients and harmful binders. Formulated with glutathione and silymarin to effectively cleanse and protect the liver.

Dandelion, scientifically known as Taraxacum officinale

Dandelion is a common weed found all over the world. It is known for its liver-cleansing properties and can be added to salads and juices. Dandelions are readily available in most markets.

This flower is quite common and possesses numerous health benefits, yet it is often labeled as a mere "weed." Its fresh leaves can be added to salads, and their strong cleansing properties make dandelion a key ingredient in detoxifying cleanses. This product is a great supporter of liver and kidney health, and it plays a crucial role in weight loss due to its low calorie content and satisfying effect.

Applications and Purpose

This product is excellent for liver health as it promotes bile production and helps with gallbladder emptying. This plant is highly effective for liver and gallbladder issues. Moreover, it can stimulate the appetite, aid in food digestion, and provide a gentle laxative effect to prevent constipation. Utilize it in natural tea, fresh salad, or a few tablespoons of fresh juice before meals. This will help with diuretic and cleansing effects, crucial for preventing water retention and eliminating calcium mineral oxalate crystals to prevent kidney stones. With its crucial role in supporting the liver organ, this makes it an effective treatment for eczema and rashes caused by autointoxication. Dandelion is a popular choice during seasonal transitions. This treatment is highly effective for curbing overeating, making it perfect for managing weight. Moreover, it functions as a poultice externally to aid in the healing of wounds and bruises.

Tips for maximizing the effectiveness of Dandelion

With its freshly picked leaves, you can create a refreshing juice using a blender or add them to a salad. If you fail to get it fresh, you can find it in troches or teabags for infusions and decoctions. Dosage options include 1/2 to 1 teaspoon (2 to 5 milliliters) every 8 hours, water extract 3/4 to 2 teaspoons (4 to 10 milliliters) every

8 hours, and pills (powdered or dry).

Dandelion Remedies

Alone

Prepare a digestive and liver organ cleansing infusion by adding a teaspoon of dandelion to a glass of boiling water. Let it steep for 10 minutes and then cool it down. Consume three mugs daily, approximately half an hour before meals. This treatment not only aids in digestion but also purifies the entire body.

Merged

Blend equal parts of liver-cleansing ingredients boldo, artichoke, dandelion, and peppermint for a hepatoprotective and diuretic infusion. Add a teaspoon of the mix to a glass of boiling water and let it steep for 10 minutes. Enjoy it as a pre-meal drink. It may support healthy digestion and help eliminate waste from the body.

Recommendations for a Mindful Lifestyle

Check out Oregon's Crazy Harvest Organic Dandelion

Root capsules!

Experience Oregon's Crazy Harvest with their authentic dandelion root powder, designed for optimal absorption and harnessing the benefits of this potent liver-cleansing ingredient. These vegan tablets make it easy to consume dandelion powder without having to deal with its bitter taste, perfect for those who are not fans of herbs.

Fumitory, also known as Fumaria officinalis

This herb is considered a sacred and somewhat mystical liver cleansing plant that can have a positive impact on your body.

The term "fumitory" originates from the Latin word "fumus" ("smoke"). It remains uncertain whether it induces tears like smoke when crushed or if its leaves simply resemble smoke from a fire. According to ancient sorcerers, burning this plant was thought to repel evil spirits.

Applications and Purpose

Its antispasmodic, diuretic, and cleansing properties are impressive, but its ability to support gallbladder function stands out the most. With its cholagogue and choleretic impact, it greatly improves the digestive process. Fumitory can help alleviate heavy and difficult digestions, migraines, and intestinal spasms. When applied externally, it proves to be a fantastic emollient for alleviating eczema and rashes.

Effective ways to utilize Fumitory

Gather it on display, let it air dry in the shade, and store it in sealed glass containers, away from light. These troches are ready to be used to make tea. You can also find it in liquid or dry form and in pills. The pill option is the most convenient as the manufacturer specifies the dose, instructions, and expiration date.

Remedies for Fumitory

Alone

For a soothing digestive infusion, simply combine 1 teaspoon of fumitory with a cup of water. Let it steep for

10 minutes and then cool it down. Sweeten it with honey or glucose, and have 3 mugs daily before meals.

Merged

Create a natural tea for gallstones by combining liver purifying foods and herbs like boldo, dandelion, peppermint, and fumitory in equal parts. Put a teaspoon of the mixture into a glass and pour in boiling water. Let it steep for 10 minutes and then cool it down. Consume three mugs daily to aid in fat digestion, eliminate toxins and bacteria, and manage gallstones.

Chapter 2

Natural Detox for Kidney and Liver

Here, we will explore six herbs that can help enhance kidney and liver function in a natural way.

1. Thistle of milk

This herb has been a staple in medicine for many years. Information indicates that Romans used it in the first century for liver health. Silymarin is the active component that supports the health of our kidneys and liver.

What are the Effects of Milk Thistle on the Kidneys?

Silymarin could potentially aid in the faster recovery of kidney cells exposed to harmful chemicals.

Milk thistle is rich in flavonoids and antioxidants, which can help boost your body's antioxidant production. Milk thistle significantly boosts the expression of genes linked to the production of three potent antioxidants in the kidneys: Glutathione, Superoxide Dismutase, and

Catalase.

Milk thistle is known for its ability to reduce inflammation in the kidneys and potentially provide protection against kidney cancer. Milk thistle's active component has been found to reduce the activity of genes that cause cancer, preventing malignant cells from multiplying efficiently.

How does Milk Thistle affect the liver?

Milk thistle stands out as one of the top natural herbs for liver detox due to its powerful impact on liver function. Here are some benefits of it: - Reducing inflammation - Stabilizing membranes in the liver - Boosting glutathione production - Increasing Superoxide Dismutase - Decreasing liver organ tumor cellular division

Furthermore, it shields your liver from damage by detoxifying toxins. Milk thistle can extend the survival time of individuals with alcohol-related liver cirrhosis!

Milk thistle affects both of our detoxification organs in a similar way. This product is our top recommendation for naturally detoxifying the kidneys and liver.

2. Marshmallow Root

Originating from a Greek word, marshmallow means "to heal." When consumed, it forms a gel-like substance and is commonly utilized for soothing sore throats. This product boasts anti-inflammatory, antibacterial, and antifungal properties. Fortunately, this herb offers significant benefits for our kidneys and liver.

What are the effects of Marshmallow root on the Kidney?

One issue that some people worry about is the development of kidney stones.

By using herbs with diuretic properties. Diuretics help increase urine production and eliminate waste through the kidneys. Marshmallow root could potentially act as a diuretic to help support a natural kidney cleanse.

What is the impact of Marshmallow root on the liver?

Marshmallow root contains polysaccharides that aid in

wound healing due to its potent antioxidant properties. Over time, the bile ducts in the liver may become damaged. Marshmallow root works to alleviate this discomfort. It actually promotes the generation of our epithelial cell. They are the cells found within your organs and ducts. Ensuring your bile duct is in good health can significantly aid your liver in the detoxification process.

Another fantastic aspect of marshmallows is their ability to bind to toxins. Eliminating toxins from the body before they can cause harm. We simply appreciate this root for its cleansing properties on the liver and kidneys.

3. Parsley

Enhance your plate at a restaurant with this vibrant green herb! This product is packed with flavonoids, vitamins, nutrients, and antioxidants. Parsley boasts potent detoxification properties for the kidneys and liver that could be advantageous for us.

What are the effects of parsley on the kidneys?

Parsley is an excellent herb for preventing kidney stones due to its diuretic properties. Among various chemicals, parsley appears to be most effective in reducing kidney stones. The scale and level of stone decreased, and the kidney cells were healthier. Parsley is a potent natural supplement for supporting kidney health.

How does parsley affect the liver?

Parsley is considered a bitter herb. Using bitter herbal products can potentially stimulate bile release, aiding in liver cleansing. Parsley is known to boost glutathione production, which plays a key role in safeguarding your liver from damage.

Parsley can also assist in reducing blood sugar levels, which can cause inflammation in the liver if elevated. It may help protect your liver by reducing inflammatory liver enzymes.

Similar to marshmallow, parsley could aid in attaching to and eliminating toxins from your body.

Parsley is known for its diuretic and protective properties, making it a great herb for kidney detoxification and liver health!

4. Gynostemma

This herb has been utilized for many years. It has earned the nickname "poor man's ginseng" due to sharing some of the same constituents as Korean ginseng. It boosts the immune system and enhances energy levels. Furthermore, it supports the detoxification of our liver and kidneys.

What are the effects of Gynostemma on the kidney?

When our organs are damaged by exposure to toxins, a process known as fibrosis can occur. Our cells end up producing scar tissue instead of healthy tissue. Scar tissue formation disrupts the normal function of tissues, hindering the kidney's ability to detoxify efficiently. Severe cases of fibrosis may result in total kidney function loss. Gynostemma has the ability to influence the genes in our kidneys, promoting the production of healthy cells and decreasing fibrosis.

What are the effects of Gynostemma on the liver?

Gynostemma offers similar benefits in reducing fibrosis in the liver as it does in the kidney. Scar tissue formation can become solid and unyielding, hindering the proper function of your liver. Exciting findings reveal that liver tissue can become leaner and severe liver fibrosis may decrease by 33% in less than eight weeks! Optimal liver cleansing can be supported by maintaining healthy tissues.

Moreover, it impacts the genes linked to the development of liver cancer cells and has demonstrated the ability to prevent their multiplication, potentially offering protection against liver cancer.

Gynostemma is a powerful anti-inflammatory for our intestines as well. The next step in your liver detox is focusing on the intestines. The liver releases toxins and bacteria into this part of your drainage system for further processing by the body. Gynostemma supports the kidneys, liver, and intestines, tripling its benefits. This is one of our top picks for enhancing your natural detoxification.

5. Beetroot

Beetroot has evolved beyond being just the vegetable you disliked as a child. These have been enjoyed for many years due to their numerous health advantages. Beets have been found in Egyptian pyramids dating back to the Dynasty period. Unintentionally, they were supporting the cleansing of their liver and kidneys by eating beets.

What are the effects of beetroot on the kidney?

Beetroot has the potential to boost your body's production of nitric oxide. Nitric oxide expands blood vessels, leading to improved circulation. This increased blood flow can potentially improve kidney function compared to when blood circulation is restricted.

Beetroot's scarlet pigment is called betanin. It can help decrease irritation and oxidative stress. Moreover, it can help safeguard your kidneys from damage.

Beetroot can help protect your kidneys from potential damage caused by antibiotics, which can sometimes lead to kidney failure. Enhancing catalase can help boost your body's natural antioxidant levels, crucial for supporting kidney detoxification. Beetroot helps in reducing proinflammatory chemicals in the kidneys as well.

How does beetroot affect the liver?

The liver is the organ responsible for protecting your body from foreign chemicals, also known as xenobiotics. Xenobiotics are everyday substances such as pesticides, environmental pollutants, and food additives that you may encounter regularly.

These substances could be carcinogenic, which is why your liver needs to deal with them promptly. Still, they can damage the liver as it neutralizes them. Beetroot is known for boosting your body's natural antioxidants to protect the liver from damage. Issues with your DNA can also be minimized.

Eliminating these foreign substances involves a process called phase II metabolism. Betanin, the red pigment, aids in neutralizing free radicals produced during the cleansing process, making it beneficial for everyone.

Beetroot, a plant that influences our genes, is worth noting. It may help downregulate the genes associated with liver cancer.

The protective pigment and gene influencing properties of beetroot, combined with our selection of natural liver and kidney detox herbs, contribute to its benefits.

6. Ginger

Ginger is considered one of the most popular spices globally due to its intense flavor. This strong natural herb is commonly used for nausea relief, while also supporting the detoxification of your liver and kidneys.

What impact does ginger have on the kidney?

Ginger can significantly enhance your kidney cleansing abilities!

Proven to increase the body's natural antioxidants in the kidneys.

- Decrease inflammation.

- Aid in eliminating toxins and bacteria in the

kidneys.

- Minimize fibrosis.

- Promote the development of healthier kidney cells.

This uncomplicated root herb is a powerhouse when it comes to kidney detoxification.

How does ginger affect the liver?

Rest assured, Ginger will not let you down when it comes to our liver organ detox.

It's unclear how ginger achieves this, but it can affect the genes related to fat production in the liver. It can assist in preventing lipid storage, which helps safeguard against fatty liver disease. When excess fat builds up in the liver, it can hinder the organ from functioning effectively. This results in fibrosis and a decrease in blood flow to the liver, leading to a significant reduction in detoxification.

Ginger swiftly reduces inflammation and supports the production of our own antioxidants.

One advantage that applies to both our liver and kidneys

is shielding against toxins. Cadmium has the ability to alter gene expression and increase the activity of cancer-related genes. Ginger has the ability to counteract this and shield you from harmful substances.

Ginger is a simple yet potent addition to your kidney and liver organ detox protocol.

Chapter 3

Detoxify Your Lungs Naturally

Steam/vapor treatment

Inhaling water vapor can help clear the airways and assist the lungs in draining mucus through vapor therapy, also known as vapor inhalation.

People with lung conditions may experience a worsening of their symptoms in cold or dry air. This weather can cause dryness in the airways and reduce blood circulation.

On the other hand, steam creates a cozy and humid environment that enhances yoga breathing and helps to thin mucus in the airways and lungs. Breathing in water vapor can quickly provide relief and make breathing easier.

A recent study with 16 male participants diagnosed with Chronic Obstructive Pulmonary Disease (COPD) revealed that steam mask therapy resulted in significantly reduced heart rates and respiratory rates compared to non-steam mask therapy.

Yet, the individuals did not report any long-term enhancements in their respiratory function.

This therapy shows promise as a short-term solution, but further research is needed to fully understand its benefits for lung health.

Master the technique of controlled coughing.

Coughing helps your body naturally get rid of toxins and bacteria trapped in mucus. Coughing helps to release excess mucus in the lungs, allowing it to be expelled through the air passages.

Doctors recommend that individuals with COPD engage in this exercise to help clear their lungs effectively.

Here are steps to help cleanse your lungs of excess mucus:

- Please sit down on the seat with your back straight, ensuring both feet are flat on the floor.

- Wrap your arms around the stomach.

- Slowly breathe in through your nostrils.

- Lean forward and exhale slowly, pressing your arms against your stomach.

- Remember to cough a few times while exhaling, with your jaws slightly open.

- Slowly breathe in through your nostrils.

- Remember to rest and repeat as needed.

Remove Mucus from Your Lungs

Positioning your body in different ways helps to clear mucus from the lungs using gravity. Engaging in this practice can enhance breathing and aid in managing or avoiding lung infections.

Postural drainage techniques vary based on the position used.

1. Behind you

- Get comfortable on the floor or a bed.

- Position cushions under the sides to ensure the chest muscles are lower than the sides.

- Slowly breathe in through your nose and breathe out through your mouth. Make sure to exhale twice as long as you inhale to achieve a 1:2 breathing ratio.

- Keep going for a few moments.

2. Tailored to suit your needs

- Rest on one side, supporting the head with an arm or pillow.

- Place cushions under the sides.

- Engage in the 1:2 yoga breathing pattern.

- Keep going for a few moments. - Alternate between the two.

3. In the vicinity of your stomach

- Arrange a variety of pillows on the floor.

- Get comfortable by lying on your stomach surrounded by pillows. Ensure the edges are kept above the chest area.

- Fold the arms under the top for support.

- Remember to practice the 1:2 respiration pattern.

- Keep going for a few moments.

4. Get moving!

Engaging in regular physical activity can enhance both physical and mental well-being while reducing the risk of various health conditions such as stroke and heart disease. Working out makes the muscles work more intensely, leading to a higher rate of breathing and more oxygen being delivered to the muscles. Moreover, it improves circulation, helping the body eliminate excess skin tightening caused by exercise. Your body will swiftly adapt to accommodate the demands of consistent physical activity. The muscles will learn to use oxygen more efficiently and reduce skin tightening.

Even though individuals with chronic lung conditions may find it challenging to exercise, they can still enjoy the benefits of regular physical activity. If you have COPD, cystic fibrosis, or asthma, it's important to consult a doctor before beginning a new exercise regimen.

5. Green tea

Green tea herb is rich in antioxidants that can help reduce inflammation in the lungs. These substances could potentially shield lung cells from the damaging effects of inhaling smoke.

According to a recent study, over 1,000 adults in Korea found that individuals who consumed a minimum of 2 cups of green tea daily showed improved lung function compared to non-drinkers.

6. Foods that help reduce inflammation

When the airways are inflamed, breathing can become challenging and the chest muscles may appear weighed down and congested. Consuming anti-inflammatory foods may help alleviate inflammation and alleviate these symptoms.

Combat inflammation with these powerful foods: - turmeric - leafy greens - cherries - blueberries - olives - walnuts - beans - lentils.

7. Performing chest percussion

Using percussion is a great method to help clear excess mucus from your lungs. Health care providers or respiratory therapists use cupped hands to rhythmically tap the chest wall to dislodge trapped mucus in the lungs.

By combining chest muscles percussion and postural drainage, you can effectively clear the airways of excess mucus.

Discover 7 natural foods and herbs to promote stronger, healthier lungs

1. Peppermint

Here's the scoop: Fresh breath not only benefits those around you but also your body. The American Cancer Society highlights the use of peppermint oil for treating lung conditions, with recent studies suggesting potential benefits for athletes' respiratory health. An Iranian study published in the Journal of the International Society of Sports Nutrition found that individuals who consumed water infused with peppermint oil showed enhanced respiratory rates, potentially attributed to the mint's ability to relax bronchial muscles.

Improving Air Quality: For inhalation, add 3 to 4 drops to tepid to warm water, as recommended by the American Cancer Society. Meanwhile, the analysis revealed a quantity of 0.05 milliliters of peppermint oil in 500 milliliters of mineral water.

2. Eucalyptus

Australia is a destination that can truly take your breath away. Eucalyptus, a plant native to the Land, has demonstrated effectiveness in preventing bronchitis flare-ups when combined with two other essential oils derived from lime and pine. This is why cough drops frequently include various components of the eucalyptus plant.

Improving Air Quality: Add a few drops of eucalyptus oil to a bowl of boiling water (create a tent with a towel over your head to trap the steam) and inhale the vapors with your eyes closed for 10 minutes. According to a report in the Decision Medicine Review, this method has been found to be effective in alleviating symptoms of respiratory infections, rhinitis, and sinusitis because of the oil's antibacterial, antiviral, and anti-inflammatory qualities.

3. Vitamin D

Individuals with a vitamin D deficiency may be at a higher risk of developing respiratory infections, as reported in Supplements & Hormones. The authors of the analysis suggest that sunlight supplementation could be a treatment for asthma.

Breathe Easier: The Institute of Medicine's Food and Nutrition Board suggests a daily intake of 600 IU of vitamin D, with a maximum recommended intake of 4,000 IU per day. Consult your healthcare provider to see if it's a good fit for you.

4. Tea

In a study involving guinea pigs, dark tea was found to prevent the harmful effects of tobacco smoke such as oxidative stress, inflammation, cell death, and lung injury. Similar to many other food sources that can improve lung health, it appears that the tea's high antioxidant content is what provides the benefits.

Improving Air Quality: Opt for black tea instead of dark espresso for a morning warm-up or a daily pick-me-up.

5. Whey protein

Can whey help improve respiratory health? One study has indicated that using whey-based supplements could potentially benefit individuals with cystic fibrosis. Whey boosts levels of glutathione, an antioxidant that protects the lungs from damage.

To Improve Air Quality: Include 10 grams of whey protein isolate in your daily diet, as indicated in the analysis, twice a day.

6. Apples

Recent report from London suggests that consuming an apple daily could help prevent lung issues. Researchers from St. George's Infirmary Medical School found that out of 2,500 participants in the study, those who consumed five or more apples per week showed a slight improvement in their overall lung function. Quercetin, an antioxidant found in apples, may offer protection to the lungs from smoke and other pollutants.

Improving Air Quality: Opt for organic apples as a late-afternoon snack to boost alertness.

7. Blueberries

Here's the scoop: Lately, there have been positive updates on blueberries, with research connecting them to enhanced heart health, improved cognitive function, and weight management. Experts have recently discovered that blueberries, with their high antioxidant content, could potentially help mitigate the negative effects of air pollution. According to a study presented at the American Heart Association's annual conference in 2014, researchers discovered that senior men who had consumed flavonoid-rich foods like blueberries were less likely to experience changes in heart function during periods of heavy smog in Boston. Chocolates and wines, while rich in flavonoids, also come with a higher calorie content that may offset their advantages. Flavonoids are believed to potentially enhance the immune system and alter gene expression to protect against environmental pollutants.

Introducing the Ultimate Lung Cleansing Juice

In addition to the suggestions above, another juice is worth trying. Start your day with a glass of water mixed with the juice of 2 lemons to boost your immune system and promote lung health. Consider using grapefruit instead of lemons. For lunch, whip up a refreshing smoothie that promotes lung health, prevents cramps, and helps with fluid balance. Enjoy multiple potassium-rich smoothies:

- *1 banana*

Ingredients needed for the recipe: - 1/2 cup of prunes - 1/2 cup of strawberries - 1/2 cup papaya - 2 cups of grain or almond milk

- *Three dates.*

For lunch or dinner, consider incorporating foods rich in carotenoids to support lung health by strengthening lung tissues and protecting cells.

Several foods are rich in carotenoids: sweet potato, butternut squash, pumpkin, cantaloupe, red peppers, grapefruit, apricots, mango, tomatoes, and papaya. Whether in a salad or a smoothie, these can be a great addition.

Lastly, before heading to bed (2 hours after eating), it's recommended to take a lung supplement along with a glass of cranberry juice. These small, black fruits boast numerous health benefits, such as antibacterial and anti-inflammatory properties that can help eliminate tar from the lungs.

Chapter 4

What is the Process for Cleaning Your Blood?

Detox has become a significant trend in the 21st century. Various programs and techniques promise to help you cleanse and detoxify your body, from diet detoxes to cleansing to blood detoxes.

After completing the detox, you should experience a boost in energy levels. Many statements lack thorough research, especially when overlooking the liver's role in blood purification.

How does the liver keep your blood clean?

Your liver is one of the largest organs in your body. Detoxifying your body is crucial.

Here's what your liver does:

- It filters your blood.

- Helps with nutrient processing.

- Eliminates toxins, such as byproducts from medication and alcohol breakdown.

Your liver contains numerous lobules. These tiny regions filter the blood and release bile to break down substances in your body.

Your liver organ eliminates toxins and bacteria in various ways, such as:

- Transforming ammonia into urea.

- Handling and eliminating excess bilirubin, a byproduct of red blood cell breakdown.

- Generating immune system cells to eradicate bacteria, potential bacteria, and toxins from your blood.

Although the liver primarily filters your blood, there are other organs in your body that also play a role in filtering.

Your lungs play a crucial role in filtering out harmful substances in the air, like toxins found in tobacco smoke.

Your intestines eliminate parasites and other unwanted

organisms.

Your kidneys filter out excess toxins, bacteria, and waste from your blood, releasing them in your urine.

Things to consider before trying any herb

Countless products in the industry market themselves as detoxifiers.

Detox Teas

Detoxification teas made from various herbs are available at health food stores and pharmacies. For example, dandelion and nettle leaf, known for their diuretic properties. Other products, like senna leaf, have a gentle laxative effect.

While these teas are quite good, their cleansing properties are probably not superior to a cup of green or black tea.

Charcoal-infused Drinks and Juices

For quite some time, doctors have been utilizing activated charcoal to minimize the absorption and effects of specific poisons in the intestines. Currently, juice and drink companies are incorporating charcoal into beverages to promote body detoxification. According to experts, charcoal can effectively bind to toxins in your digestive system, helping to reduce the amount of harmful substances that can enter your bloodstream.

Yet, there isn't a substantial body of research supporting the benefits of adding charcoal to beverages. No scientific evidence supports the claim that charcoal is particularly effective in detoxifying your blood or promoting overall health. Many individuals who drink these beverages claim to feel more energized during physical activity, although not everyone may notice a difference.

For more information on medications that may interact or lose effectiveness when taken with activated charcoal, visit the Mayo Clinic website. Activated charcoal is not recommended if you have a history of gastrointestinal bleeding, recent surgery, or indigestion. It is possible to consume too much activated charcoal. It is advisable to consult your doctor before ingesting activated charcoal.

The FDA does not approve or regulate activated charcoal or other natural remedies.

Detox Diets

Detox diets have been around for quite some time. These diets usually involve a strict eating plan to purify your blood and usually aim to help you lose weight. Detox diets typically remove substances like alcohol, caffeine, and gluten.

Red meat and processed sugars, among others.

Certain detox diets may encourage better food choices. Some diets can be quite limiting, like juice detox or other restrictive eating plans that eliminate certain foods and beverages in order to boost energy levels.

Since the body is capable of eliminating toxins on its own, there is no need for a strict diet plan. Embracing a nutritious diet rich in fruits, vegetables, lean meats, and whole grains can be beneficial.

Protecting Your Liver

Given the significance of your liver in purifying your blood, it's crucial to take steps to protect it. Fortunately, several routine healthy habits can assist in maintaining the liver's health. Here are a few suggestions:

Make sure to get vaccinated against Hepatitis A and B as they are viral infections that can harm your liver.

• Keeping a healthy weight is important: Holding excess fat can lead to a condition known as non-alcoholic fatty liver disease. Eating nutritious foods and exercising regularly are key to managing your weight.

When getting tattoos or body piercings, always make sure to check the shop's cleaning practices to avoid sharing or using contaminated needles.

Make sure to practice safe sex to lower your risk of contracting sexually transmitted infections like hepatitis B or C.

• Pay attention to the recommendations provided on your medications: It's crucial to avoid alcohol when your medication's label advises against it.

Avoid consuming too much alcohol. Your liver filters the body systems and detoxifies alcohol consumption along with many other products. Excessive alcohol consumption can lead to scarring and damage to liver cells.

Steer clear of using illegal substances: Your liver filters out harmful byproducts from medication consumption. Regular use can result in serious damage to your liver, especially when combined with alcohol.

Chapter 5

Eight foods that are necessary for blood purification are natural blood purifiers.

Your blood is responsible for several bodily functions, such as maintaining the flow of blood throughout your body and transporting oxygen, hormones, carbohydrates, fats, and cells to your immune system. Our bodies constantly accumulate microorganisms and toxins from various food sources, environmental pollution, and stress, among other things. The act of washing strengthens your body's resistance to disease, improves the quality of your skin, and controls physiological changes. While your blood is being purified by your liver, kidneys, and lungs. Generally speaking, some foods will ease the process somewhat. I want to draw your attention to the following reasons why cleansing and detoxifying the blood is so important:

- You'll become less susceptible to skin conditions that are indicative of blood impurities, such as acne, pimples, and dry, unhealthy skin.

- Blood purification also lessens the risk of several illnesses and skin disorders like allergies, migraines, nausea, and so on that are brought on by tainted blood.

- The functions of the major organs are impacted by healthy blood flow. The lymphatic system, lungs, liver, heart, and kidneys all benefit from a healthy blood count.

- Blood cleansing is necessary to ensure that gases, such as air and skin tightening, are continuously transported to and from the lungs and all other bodies.

- Your pH level, water balance, and temperature are all significantly regulated by the blood purification procedure.

- White blood cells, which help minimize blood loss following an accident and ensure a healthy platelet count, are present in healthy blood.

The following foods may help to stimulate the process of blood purification:

1. Kale

One of the best natural blood purifiers that can help rid your body of toxins and bacteria is broccoli, according to reports. This vegetable is rich in calcium, phosphate, manganese, potassium, diet fiber, vitamin C, and omega-3 fatty acids. Frequent use of broccoli guarantees the onset of antioxidants that aid in blood detoxification and enhance the body's ability to fight sickness. Toss it into your salads; you must include it in your regular foods.

2. Ripe Fruits

Pectin fiber, found in fruits including apples, guavas, pears, and plums, aids in blood purification. They do more than just attach to extra fat in your blood; they also tie to poisons and other dangerous compounds, which they can effectively expend and eliminate. In addition, tomatoes' lycopene glutathione helps flush out waste and toxins. Remember to include a small amount of berries, such as blackberries, cranberries, and strawberries, in your daily diet to support the health of your liver organs.

3. Vegetables with green leaves

Green leafy vegetables may not be to your taste, but why not tell you that they are packed with important nutrients and antioxidants that help ward against illness? To ensure healthy blood flow, choose among mustard greens, kale, lettuce, and spinach. These greens are responsible for enhancing the liver's enzymes, which support the blood cleansing process.

4. Beets

According to reports, beetroot is a natural source of nitrates and antioxidant betalains, which might lessen liver damage and inflammation. The majority of research also demonstrate that beetroot juice increases the body's natural detoxifying enzyme production. Incorporate beetroot into your salad.

5. Jaggery

An all-natural blood purifier, used in Indian households primarily for its glucose substitute, these raw sugars contain fiber that aids in digestive system cleansing, constipation prevention, and waste removal from the body. Jaggery's high iron content promotes healthy blood flow throughout the body and aids in the restoration of hemoglobin levels. Additionally, it may remove clots from your blood, which would help your blood become even cleaner.

6. H2O

One of the most popular and straightforward natural blood cleansers is water. Your kidneys need urine to remove toxins and bacteria from your blood, so drinking water is typically a better chance to significantly support this process. Water helps your organs function properly and flushes out all of the toxins and dangerous chemicals that are inside of you. Ayurvedic blood purification is best achieved by storing hot water in a copper jar overnight and drinking it the next day with a clear stomach. The extra effort your liver must perform to purify your blood will be cooled by the copper, and water will speed up the process of expelling waste.

7. Ginger

One of the finest natural remedies for reducing inflammation is definitely turmeric. It might enhance the function of the liver. Its curcumin content may be the solution to some of our body's issues. The majority of specialists recommend turmeric dairy since it not only provides your body with vital nutrients but also acts as a health tonic and generates red blood cells.

8. Lemon

Warm water with lemon is generally thought to encourage the burning of extra fat and reduce the possibility of renal strain since the vitamins and minerals in the lemons aid in blood and body detoxification.

Keep including these necessary nutrients in your diet to ensure that your blood system is healthy and pure.

Using Foods, Herbs, and Other Natural Remedies to Clean Your Blood

There are three primary purposes for the arteries:

• **_Regulation:_** Your blood plays a vital role in controlling your body's temperature, pH, and drinking water balance. Many vital functions are carried out by your blood, so it seems sense that people would want to know how to keep pollutants, toxins, and bacteria out of their blood.

Thankfully, your body already has all it needs to carry out the detoxification process and eliminate waste from the blood—more precisely, the kidneys and liver organ.

• **_Transport:_** The blood carries nutrients and gasses, such as oxygen, to and through the lungs and other parts of your body. The blood also carries waste, physical hormones, and other cells, as well as nutrients from your digestive system to any or all other parts of your body.

• **_Protection:_** The blood has platelet factors to coagulate the blood and reduce blood loss from a personal injury, as well as white blood cells to destroy invasive germs.

• **_Liver:_** Located in the upper right portion of the stomach is the liver organ. It is advantageous to turn food into energy. Additionally, it transforms bacteria and toxins— such as alcohol, poisons, and medications—into safe compounds and guarantees that they may be eliminated from your body.

• **_Kidneys:_** The kidneys are two organs that resemble beans that filter blood and eliminate waste.

The lymphatic system, spleen, intestines, and skin are all involved in your body's natural detoxification process.

You will come across a great deal of false information regarding purging and cleaning products that purport to clean and purify the blood. There is no indication that the components in these supplements instantly remove waste, toxins, or bacteria from the blood; instead, they can benefit the blood indirectly by supporting the function of the kidney and liver organs.

Top Foods for a Holistic Cleanse

No miraculous diet exists that can help with blood purification. A standard healthy diet rich in fruits and vegetables is a great place to start.

Additional foods that have been shown to have a good

impact on the liver's and kidneys' capacity to remove waste and toxins from the blood include:

Water

Getting adequate water into your diet is by far the best strategy to enhance the function of your kidneys. Water plays a major role in your kidneys' ability to eliminate waste products from your body. In order for blood to flow freely, water also keeps your arteries open. Nephrotoxicity can result from extreme dehydration.

Throughout the day, your urine should be colorless or pale yellow. The American Kidney Association recommends that an individual should be generating approximately six cups of urine daily.

A sufficient amount of water to drink varies for each individual. Eight glasses of water a day is a general recommendation, but you may require more if you engage in vigorous exercise or if you take additional factors into consideration. In general, males require more water than females.

Cruciferous Vegetables: Brussels sprouts, cauliflower, broccoli, and cabbage

People with renal illness are often advised to eat cruciferous vegetables. They are quite healthful and high in antioxidants. It has been demonstrated by Trusted Source that they lower the risk of kidney cancer among other cancers. They are also quite adaptable. They can be eaten raw, steamed, cooked, grilled, or combined with other ingredients to make a soup or casserole.

Berries

Antioxidants found in high concentration in blueberries may shield the liver from harm. According to research conducted on pets, Trusted Source, whole blueberries can assist maintain the liver's health.

You can consume fresh or frozen blueberries, or you can add them to smoothies, porridge, or yogurt.

Cranberries

It is common for cranberries to be marketed as having advantages for the urinary tract. Their ability to deter bacteria from adhering to the urinary tract has already been demonstrated, protecting your kidneys from illness.

All it takes to benefit from the fruits' benefits is to add a few fresh cranberries to salads, smoothies, and cereal.

Coffee

Coffee consumption may have protective effects in the vicinity of the liver. According to studies published in Reliable Source, coffee consumption may also lessen the risk of liver organ cancer in those with chronic liver disease by reducing the likelihood of cirrhosis.

In patients with chronic liver disease, espresso is linked to a lower risk of death and, in those with hepatitis C, an improved prophylactic response to antiviral therapy. Coffee's ability to prevent the accumulation of excess fat and collagen in the liver may be the cause of these enormous advantages.

Garlic

Any meal benefits greatly from the flavor that garlic, whether raw or powdered, brings. They may lower blood pressure and cholesterol because they have anti-inflammatory qualities. It's recommended to keep blood pressure in check because elevated blood pressure can damage renal arteries.

Grapefruit

Antioxidants included in grapefruit may help reduce edema in the body. The majority of research on the effects of grapefruit's constituents has already been done on animals, but the results are encouraging.

According to these research published in Trusted Source, grapefruit's antioxidants may be able to shield the liver from harm as well as the harmful effects of alcohol.

Apples

Apples include a significant quantity of pectin, a type of dietary fiber. Your blood sugar is regulated by soluble fiber. Whatever keeps blood sugar in check should have a favorable, indirect impact on kidney health because high blood sugar might harm your kidneys. Apples are a great snack, especially when combined with a tiny bit of peanut butter.

Fish

Certain seafood varieties, such as tuna, sardines, and salmon, are high in omega-3 fatty acids. Omega-3 fatty acids have been shown to lower blood pressure and blood triglyceride levels, which may help your kidneys and liver.

Keep in mind that seafood has a high protein content. You should consume less high-protein foods if you currently have renal disease. Consuming too much protein will increase the workload on your kidneys.

Herbal Remedies for the Liver and Kidney Organs

Numerous herbs are beneficial to health. That being said, you should refrain from ingesting high concentrations of natural extracts since they may be hazardous to your kidneys. If you currently have liver or renal illness, you should avoid using any herbs. Before making any changes to your daily eating regimen or product plan, speak with your doctor.

Ginger

Ginger may help your body better regulate blood sugar. Similarly, research has indicated that ginger may be useful in the treatment of nonalcoholic fatty liver disease (NAFLD). You can drink ginger like a tea or add it to some foods as a taste enhancer.

Green tea: Research indicates that ingesting green tea herb may help to strengthen the liver, lower excess fat in the liver, and maybe prevent liver cancer. The greatest advantages have been found in those who consume four (4) glasses or more per day.

Roselle (Hibiscus)

A kind of hibiscus with a cranberry-like flavor is called roselle. It has been demonstrated to have diuretic effects on the body and may help with renal filtration. There is hibiscus tea available. You can add the calyces to your salads if you're fortunate enough to grow this flower in your own backyard garden.

Parsley

Parsley may also strengthen and shield the liver, according to research on cats. According to another study, it may aid in urine production, which aids in the kidneys' waste removal. You can keep doing this and garnish a variety of dishes, particularly Italian fare, with fresh parsley.

Dandelion

Because dandelion has diuretic properties, it increases the amount of water that passes through your kidneys. As such, it can assist in removing waste from your blood. Furthermore, according to some recent research, dandelion may be the greatest herb for liver organ performance. Making tea from the leaves, flowers, or roots of dandelion is unquestionably the greatest method to enjoy this herb.

Chapter 6

5 Effective Herbs to Naturally Detoxify Your Blood and How to Prepare Them.

The liver, known as the body's detoxifying organ, filters blood continuously to remove any chemicals or toxins that may have entered your bloodstream. How about providing some assistance? Herbs for blood cleansing help remove toxins and bacteria from your lymph system, kidneys, and liver, promoting pure blood circulation to all your organs.

These five herbs are commonly found and are effective in cleansing your blood and aiding in overall detoxification to boost your health.

1. Burdock Root

Burdock is renowned for its blood-cleansing properties and is considered a top herb for pores and skin. It helps eliminate toxins and bacteria from your body by supporting the liver and lymphatic system. Burdock is recognized for its diuretic properties and its ability to support the kidneys in filtering out pollutants from the blood. This nutrient-rich root is excellent for boosting blood health and fortifying the entire body.

Ways to make the most of it:

Burdock is versatile and can be enjoyed in various forms like pills, liquid extracts, tinctures, or tea. You can find this edible root in the fresh produce section of the local health store. Enhance it by adding more fresh vegetables or incorporating it into soups.

2. Dandelion

Rich in phytonutrients and numerous antioxidants, this herbal plant can help remove toxins from your digestive system and blood, while also fighting free radicals. Dandelion helps the liver and pancreas capture toxins in the blood and purify it.

Ways to make the most of it:

To enjoy the detoxifying benefits of dandelion, simply brew a tea using fresh or dried dandelion leaves, plants, or root.

3. Reishi Mushroom

This herb is a Chinese tonic known for boosting the liver's cleansing process. Reishi mushroom contains ganoderic acid, which acts as an antihistamine and helps reduce inflammation. Furthermore, it enhances the utilization of oxygen in the blood, thereby enriching it. The mushroom contains triterpenes and ganodosterone, which help protect the liver from damage by acting as antihepatotoxic agents. Additionally, it has been demonstrated to stimulate the regeneration of liver cells in individuals with advanced hepatitis.

Ways to make the most of it:

Bring 2 teaspoons of dried mushrooms to a boil in one cup of water. Let it simmer for two to three minutes, then enjoy once it has cooled down. Another great idea is to add powdered mushroom to your soups.

4. Basil

This culinary herb is widely recognized for its antibacterial and anti-inflammatory properties. Basil has a remarkable ability to cleanse your blood and eliminate any toxins from your liver and kidneys. Basil is a fantastic diuretic that helps remove toxins and bacteria from your body through urine.

Instructions for use:

Enhance your soups, salads, or pasta with 5 to 6 basil leaves for a burst of flavor and detoxifying properties. For a homemade all-natural tea, steep six to eight basil leaves in a glass of warm water.

5. Red Clover

These lovely lilac blossoms are excellent at purifying the blood and enhancing the circulatory system. Additionally, it improves blood circulation by preventing clot formation. Red clover is recognized for its anti-tumor properties and is widely trusted by herbalists worldwide, including Dr. Sebi, as a treatment for cancer.

Instructions for use:

Brew a calming and cleansing red clover tea by using three to four fresh blossoms or 1 tsp of crushed dried flowers in a cup of warm water for 10 minutes. Sip when chilled. Ready-to-use teabags and pills are available for purchase online.

Acknowledgements

Behold the magnificent triumph of this extraordinary book, a testament to the divine intervention of God Almighty and the unwavering love and support of my cherished Family, devoted Fans, avid Readers, loyal Customers, and dear Friends. Their ceaseless encouragement has paved the way for this resounding success.

www.ingramcontent.com/pod-product-compliance
Lightning Source LLC
Chambersburg PA
CBHW031133020426
42333CB00012B/358